CLINICAL INTEGRATION

Accountable Care and Population Health

Third Edition

Chapter 8. Coordinating Care – Transforming the Delivery Process

by

Michael G. Hunt, DO, FACOP, FAAP, MMI

Colleen Swedberg, MSN, RN, CNL

BOOK EXECUTIVE EDITORS

Ken Yale | Thomas Raskauskas |
Joanne Bohn | Colin Konschak

CONVURGENT
PUBLISHING

This publication is intended to provide accurate and authoritative information in regard to the subject matter covered. The statements and opinions expressed in this chapter are those of the authors.

ISBN-13: 9780991234561
ISBN-10: 0991234561

Convurgent Publishing, LLC
4445 Corporation Lane, Suite #227
Virginia Beach, VA 23462
Phone: (877) 254-9794, Fax: (757) 213-6801
Web Site: www.convurgent.com
E-mail: info@convurgent.com

Special Orders.
Bulk Quantity Sales.
Special discounts are available on quantity purchases. Please contact sales@convurgent.com.
Library of Congress Control Number: 2014959540
Bibliographic data:

Chapter 8. Coordinating Care – Transforming the Delivery Process, In: Accountable Care and Population Health, Third Edition. Chapter 8 Authors: Michael Hunt and Colleen Swedberg.

p. cm.
1. Clinical integration. 2. Clinically integrated networks. 3. Healthcare reform. 4. Health information technology. 5. Clinical quality. 6. Care coordination. 7. Behavioral health. 8. Population health.
ISBN:9780991234561

ABOUT THIS CHAPTER

This chapter manuscript represents a final draft chapter to be incorporated in the forthcoming 3rd Edition of, *Clinical Integration. Accountable Care and Population Health*. The final version of this chapter will be subject to final revisioning by its authors and editing and copyediting by the executive editors and the publisher.

ABOUT THE CHAPTER 8 AUTHORS

Michael G. Hunt, DO, FACOP, FAAP, MMI, graduated from the University of Osteopathic Medicine and Health Sciences, Des Moines, Iowa and completed his internship and residency in Pediatrics at William Beaumont Army Medical Center in 1994. After residency, he held several leadership positions including Chief of Medicine and Chief of Pediatrics. In 2005 he joined Mercy, Oklahoma City, to grow his pediatric practice. He advocated for the system to implement an EMR. His participation as physician champion and CMIO helped the organization to implement EPIC in 29 hospitals and 200 ambulatory offices representing more than 50 medical specialties.

Dr. Hunt completed his Masters in Medical Informatics at Northwestern University in 2012, and is an associate professor of informatics at St. Louis University. He is Board Certified in Pediatrics, and is an Assistant Professor of Pediatrics at St. Vincent's Hospital and Medical Center and the Frank H. Netter MD School of Medicine at Quinnipiac University. In addition to his current role as CMO/CMIO of St. Vincent's Health Partners, Inc, Dr. Hunt continues to see patients at St. Vincent's Family Health Center.

St. Vincent's Health Partners, a Physician Hospital Organization in Connecticut, is soon to be nationally recognized as a clinically integrated network by URAC Accreditation. St. Vincent's Health Partners' (SVHP) membership consists of more than 350 providers, and St. Vincent's Medical Center. The organization's mission is to be the leader in healthcare reform, provide patients with high quality cost-effective patient-centric care, and celebrate and reinforce the patient-physician relationship while respecting each participating member's desire to remain independent.

Colleen Swedberg MSN, RN, CNL, obtained her undergraduate nursing degree at the University of Calgary in Alberta, Canada, and Master of Science in Nursing at Fairfield University in Fairfield, CT. She is certified as a Clinical Nurse Leader (CNL) with the American Association of Colleges of Nursing (AACN). She worked in surgical trauma in Calgary and surgical oncology at Tulane Medical Center in New Orleans as well as community health with Tulane's hospital based home care agency, primarily in the 9th ward of New Orleans. From 1989 to 1996 Colleen worked in rural and urban programs in Haiti primarily in women and children's health including providing technical assistance to an immunization outreach project, reviewing child survival activities funded by a U.S. government grant (micronutrients, diarrhea, health education, immunizations) and with Save the Children Federation, developing the reproductive health subsector with local government and agency medical staff. In the U.S. Colleen became team leader of a VNS maternal child health program in CT, coordinating home-based skilled care to antenatal, postpartum, premature and normal maternal/newborn duos, working to improve access of a medically underserved population to community health services. In 2004, Colleen joined the team of the first Connecticut branch of a national home health care agency, Bayada Home Health Care, progressing to the clinical lead in 2007 of over 30 multidisciplinary field staff providing skilled services to acutely ill patients at home. Currently Colleen serves as Director for Care Coordination and Integration at St. Vincent's Health Partners in Bridgeport, CT. SVHP is a physician-hospital organization representing more than 350 physicians and providers, and a community medical center. SVHP is supporting the efforts of the member medical professionals and institutions to realize the Triple Aim: provide quality care that exceeds patient expectation, improve the health of the patient population, and reduce the cost-of-care. Redefining the roles of care coordination and case management and integrating the use of an organizational Playbook are key strategies to effectively provide health management of the population.

TABLE OF CONTENTS

Chapter 8. Care Coordination- Transforming the Delivery Process

Michael G. Hunt, DO, FACOP, FAAP, MMI

Colleen Swedberg, MSN, RN, CNL

Alone we can do so little; together we can do so much.(Keller, 2013)

Helen Keller
American Author
1880-1968

CHAPTER 8 LEARNING OBJECTIVES

✓ Exposure to new Care Coordination models resulting from healthcare reform.

✓ Understand how Care Coordination facilitates organizational achievement of the "Triple Aim".

✓ Exposure to a systematic approach to identifying care coordination challenges.

✓ Understand the symbiosis of Clinical Integration and Care Coordination.

✓ Understand how Care Coordination is a component of medical management and its effect on population health management.

Overview

The purpose of care coordination is to improve the health of each member of a population, assist a provider network's delivery of care to reflect quality and appropriate access that help determine the patient's experience, and collaborate with provider network participants to decrease and control the costs of healthcare for consumers and patients served by the network. This purpose reflects the goals of the "Triple Aim".(Beasley, 2009)

Care coordination should be the driving force to help manage the member population at large while engaging local healthcare resources to "manage" patient care. Care coordination is the foundation of medical management that oversees the entire population, or a specific population subset, attributed to an organization. This function within each clinically integrated network (CIN) and accountable care organization (ACO) focuses attention on standardization of processes to assure efficient patient care transitions among providers and sites of care and meeting the medical care requirements for both chronic and preventative care. Care coordination serves a central role in monitoring the population at-large and empowering local facilities, especially the primary care provider, in case managing the patient locally. The successful maturation of care coordination is critical when organization take on full risk with payor contracts.

Both care coordination and case management are mutually exclusive professional roles while being interdependent. Case management should occur directly with the patient while medical services are rendered (ED, inpatient, ambulatory service center). Case management functions best when local team members bring into play the relationship between the physician (provider) and the patient. Localized case management is positioned to activate a complete treatment plan using the most current medically relevant information.

INSIGHT: The model differentiates care coordination at the enterprise level and case management at the most local level. Case management exploits the patient provider relationship fully, where care coordination manages the population at-large and is reliant on effective case management locally!

As a function of clinically integrated services case management may include education, treatment, referral, and other clinical services (coordination and scheduling of services, facilitation and confirmation of medical information transfer (portability), and resolves actual and perceived patient barriers to continuous care). The case manager directly interacts with the patient. Care coordination may include coordination of medical activities, medical information portability, and resolution of patient/facility barriers when case management needs additional resources. Care Coordination (at the enterprise level) institutionalizes and enculturates standardized processes for patient care and collaboration, monitors the population at large, facilitates individual care, and supplements case management activities when necessary from the enterprise level. Care coordination is the macro healthcare controller, while case management manages healthcare issues at the individual patient level. Care coordination requires continuous communication with case managers and medical professionals, access to "real-time" medical information that is portable, and guides local facilities to optimize workflow and patient out-reach.

Access to highly developed diagnostic tests and interventions, delivered in state-of-the-art institutions that are not connected, contributes to duplication of effort and an expensive health care system in the U.S.(National Quality Forum, 2010) There is a perception that more sophisticated or a greater number of interventions equates to better health care. Public education about the need to understand outcomes and cost has lagged behind promotion of advances in science and technology. As a result, healthcare in the United States is intricate, highly specialized, over utilized, and expensive.

Yet while care may be delivered in a technically correct fashion within various specialties, the intricacies and specialization have led to fragmentation, in which one clinical provider often does not know what another is doing with the same patient.(National Quality Forum, 2013) Further, the complexity of care today is such that patients frequently do not understand how to care for themselves after they leave the clinical setting, even following a simple primary care visit. This situation creates a dangerous, unnecessarily complicated, and bewildering environment for patients—putting at risk of harm the very people the system seeks to serve, with sometimes disastrous consequences.(National Quality Forum, 2010)

In fact, fragmentation is a characteristic of the U.S. health care system. The system is designed to provide care and services to individuals and help them survive an episodic acute illness event.(Robinson, 2010) Multiple, specialized providers care for people with chronic illnesses. Chronic care for a single illness is often provided without knowledge of medications and care given by other specialty providers.(Reuben, 2007) Ball et. al. describes the context as systems, structures and processes that have evolved over time and have been cobbled together with unaligned assumptions in each silo.(Ball, Merry, & Verlaan-Cole L, 2013) Patients move from silo to silo within the system. A lack of coordination gives rise to 'misuse, over use, [and] underuse' of resources.(Chassin & Galvin, 1998)

Ideally, the health care system should be designed to interface with people so as to make it possible for them to have the care they need and want, can understand that care, and can assume communication occurs between providers. Various models, approaches, processes and interventions have emerged over time to address the gaps in communication and coordination inherent in the current system. These efforts are mostly band aids trying to patch a broken system rather than designs that have developed systematically and organically and can be validated and replicated, to improve value and quality outcomes with the appropriate use of data.

More than a decade ago the IOM published a landmark study, *Crossing the Quality Chasm –a New Healthcare System for the Twenty First Century* which served as a trumpet call for revamping the U.S. health care system.(Committee on Quality of Healthcare in America & Institute of Medicine, 2001) It is frequently referenced in the medical literature, programming, and academia. The study calls for improvements in six dimensions of health care performance: safety, effectiveness, patient-centeredness, timeliness, efficiency, and equity; and it asserts that those improvements cannot be achieved within the constraints of the existing system of care. It provides a rationale and a framework for the redesign of the U.S. health care system at four levels: patients' experiences; the "microsystems" that actually give care; the organizations that house and support microsystems; and the environment of laws, rules, payment, accreditation, and professional training that shape organizational action.(Berwick, 2002) These microsystems and the organizations that house them are fertile ground for care coordination.

Response to the IOM mandate to redesign the health care system is emerging, with coordination of care at the center. For example, the American Hospital Association in a 2011 presentation to its membership addressed the health care landscape, suggesting a shift is required from the volume based 'first curve' economics with stand-alone acute inpatient hospitals, to a value-based 'second curve' economics system, including realigned incentives, partnerships with shared risk, IT utilization for population management and increased coordination.(American Hospital Association, 2011)

Health reform laws, mainly the Patient Protection and Affordable Care Act of 2010 (ACA), is a defining moment in addressing the deficiencies outlined in the Quality Chasm report. The ACA targets realigning providers' financial incentives, encouraging more efficient organization and delivery of health care, and investing in preventive and population health – all elements of care coordination. Provisions in the ACA extend health insurance coverage to 32 million uninsured Americans, potentially improving access to care and equity but making care coordination even more important as the ranks of insured seeking care swell.(Davis, June 23, 2010) The legislation encourages new delivery models, such as ACOs, CINs, medical homes, health homes, and transitional care interventions, that offer incentives to providers for coordinating and improving care for chronically ill populations.(Volland,

Schraeder, Shelton, & Hess, 2012) The American Recovery and Reinvestment Act included approximately $19 billion to expand the use of health information technology – another key element in coordination of care.

Defining Care Coordination

Health care coordination, in its simplest form, involves providers, patients, and other caregivers working together to deliver health care services. In context of the ACA and new government regulations, it is also designed to meet the "Triple Aim" of improved quality, lowered costs and better patient satisfaction.

The healthcare industry and health professionals have not solidified a concept or single definition for care coordination. Many have incorrectly equated collaboration with coordination. Stille et al distinguish between care coordination and collaboration, noting that care coordination is not synonymous with collaborative care, which is simply the act of working together.(Stille, Jerant, Bell, Meltzer, & Elmore, 2005) By contrast, coordination according to Stille involves the regulation of participants to produce higher-order functioning and involves the integration of inputs from multiple entities towards a common goal. Care coordination is sometimes thought of as case management, but there are differences here too. Understanding these differences can help further define care coordination.

Not surprisingly, given the complexity and fragmentation of the healthcare system, coordination of care is the 'subject du jour' in health care redesign discussions. 'Coordination' is generally defined as the process of organizing people, groups or things in order to make them work together effectively.(Macmillan Dictionary, 2013)

Various nationally recognized health quality organizations have defined 'care coordination'. For example, the National Quality Forum (NQF) defines care coordination as "a function that helps ensure that the patient's needs and preferences for health services and information sharing across people, functions, and sites are met over time."(National Quality Forum, 2006) This definition is purposely patient-centric, does not even specify providers or organizations, and adds a time element. NQF elaborates on this definition by emphasizing information-rich, patient and patient-centered characteristics and the purposeful intention to deliver the right care to the right patient at the right time. NQF refers to care coordination as a function that allows communication across settings and between episodes of care to limit medical errors, reduce costs, and limit the pain a patient bears from care plans not integrated to meet the patient's unique needs. Further, arising from the work of the NQF and the National Priorities Partnership, care coordination is described as ensuring that patients' needs and preferences for healthcare services are understood and that they are shared as patients move from one healthcare setting to another or to home, as care is transferred from one healthcare organization to another or is shared among primary care professional and specialists.(National Priorities Partnership, 2008)

The federal government Agency for Healthcare Research and Quality (AHRQ) defines care coordination as,

> ...the deliberate organization of patient care activities between two or more participants (including the patient) involved in a patient's care to facilitate the appropriate delivery of health care services. Organizing care involves the marshalling of personnel and other resources needed to carry out all required patient care activities and is often managed by the exchange of information among participants responsible for different aspects of care."(Agency for Healthcare Research and Quality, 2011)

Care coordination here is a brokering of services for patients to ensure that needs are met and services are not duplicated by professionals participating in the same patient care. This definition does specify health professionals and others involved, including the patient, and references "other resources," which alludes to community and social services, reflecting the close relationship of this agency to government Public Health Services. AHRQ further elaborates its concept of care coordination through supporting information sharing across providers, patients, and types and levels of service, sites and time frames.

Care coordination and case management have also been used interchangeably within healthcare. For example, the Case Management Society of America defines case management as a collaborative process of assessment, planning, facilitation, care coordination, evaluation, and advocacy for options and services to meet an individual's and family's comprehensive health needs through communication and available resources to promote quality, cost-effective outcomes.(Case Management Society of America, 2013) The National Coalition on Care Coordination defines care coordination as,

> ...a client-centered, assessment-based interdisciplinary approach to integrating health care and social support services in which an individual's needs and preferences are assessed, a comprehensive care plan is developed, and services are managed and monitored by an identified care coordinator following evidence-based standards of care".(National Coalition on Care Coordination, 2013)

In this definition the two roles do not appear to be distinct.

Table 8-1 compares and contrasts the proposed care coordination concept and literature-defined case management roles. SVHP Transition Leadership Team Presentation June 5, 2014, St. Vincent's Medical Center.

Table 8-1. Comparison Between Care Coordination and Case Management

Category	Care Coordination	Case Management
Targeted Population	Organizational attributed patients	Individual patient
Education and outreach (inform and motivate	Primary: Organizational Providers Secondary: Patient	Patient
Disease Management	Oversees organizational care delivery success	Provides care for the patient
Communication	Organizational and	Individual patient and

Category	Care Coordination	Case Management
	individual members	care team
Goals	Network directed	Patient/Payer/facility directed
Care Delivery	Population management	Medical service and individual care management
Processes	System standardization	Process and implementation focused
Relationship	Primary – Local healthcare team Secondary - Patient	Primary - Patient Secondary – Local healthcare team
Network Resource	Utilize network	Utilize individual clinician
Use of Health Information Technology	Primary – Network and population management Secondary – Patient/Practice/Panel	Primary - Patient/Practice/Panel Secondary – Network and population management
Measure of Success	Population outcomes	Patient outcomes

These roles and the professionals that occupy them have significant impact on the delivery of population health management services and each organization's ability to operationalize them to effect patient care. These roles are distinctly unique, although in practice there is overlap, and have different foundational processes in the delivery of healthcare services for the population served. Notice the categories and how each role is differentiated. This chapter elaborates on these categories and what they mean for the effective delivery of health care services for CINs and ACOs.

Case management identifies appropriate providers and facilities throughout the continuum of care, ensuring that available resources are used timely and cost-effectively. Case management functions better when the environment allows direct communication between the case manager, client, and healthcare provider. The Commission for Case

Manager Certification's premise is that "...everyone benefits when clients reach their optimum level of wellness, self-management, and functional capability."(Commission for Case Management Certification, 2013) Case management facilitates wellness and autonomy through advocacy, assessment, planning, communication, education, resource management, and service facilitation. All intervention is based on the needs and values of the client.

The Library of Medicine defines case management as a traditional term for the activities that a physician or other health care professional normally performs to ensure the coordination of the medical services required by a patient.(Slee, Slee, & Schmidt, 2008) The definition of case management includes the activities of evaluating the patient, planning treatment, referral, and follow-up so that care is continuous and comprehensive and payment for the care is obtained.

Improving Chronic Illness Care's website describes care coordination as a "deliberate organization of patient care activities between two or more participants involved to facilitate the delivery of health care services".(Improving Chronic Care (ICC), 2013) Consequently, the providers managing a patient's care share clinical information and have clear, shared expectations about the patient's needs and their role in providing care. By supporting and managing the transition between participants, the patient's receipt of medical care is enhanced. Care coordination engages families during care plan development and "manages" care expectations.

Improving Chronic Illness Care website delineates the principles of care coordination to include: accessibility, individualization, family alignment, promotion of solutions to systemic problems, and attention to outcome.(Improving Chronic Care (ICC), 2013) It describes effective care coordination to be activities which promote:

- Continuous evaluation of community and environmental resources (community programs, community agencies, resource guide, relationship building with program/agency staff, develop coalitions),

- Utilization of screening tools reflective of different conditions,

- Performing needs assessment (interview family for needs, strengths, and resources),

- Development of individual family support plans (review patient needs with the family), and

- Implementing and monitoring patient care plans, and revise the plan as needed.(Improving Chronic Care (ICC), 2013)

The Commission for Case Manager Certification (CCMC) states that care coordination falls within the domain of a case manager. When looking at healthcare organization operationalization of care coordination, many institutions define care coordination as a function performed by a case manager and not as a unique professional role.(Commission for Case Management Certification, 2013) This cacophony of definitions and perspectives highlights the fragmentation of the industry and how each professional group defines care coordination to their benefit.

Models of Care Coordination versus Case Management

In 2011, the Institute for Healthcare Improvement published a white paper detailing potential care coordination models.(Institute for Healthcare Improvement, 2011) The first model was led by a nurse with support from a case manager, behaviorist, elder worker, and others to coordinate care between direct care providers; assure appropriate and timely access to services, pharmaceuticals, and durable medical equipment; teach, coach, and develop self-management strategies for chronic and acute illness, and mental health problems; and promote optimal primary care home management. The intensity of patient contact was tiered. The care coordination activities were stratified into three levels. The third level is development of a comprehensive treatment plan incorporating family dynamics, understanding long-term diverse resource requirements to facilitate continuous patient care, and facilitating continual communication between providers to effectively manage the patient's ongoing medical needs. Attention to quality metrics and organizational outcome metrics is required to justify the intensity of intervention and level of resource utilization.

In another model, Tufts Health Plan attempts to change behaviors and align economic incentives by coordinating care and focus on cost and quality care through promotion of effective settings that use care management to engage plan members and providers. The National Institutes of Health has also published data detailing case management outcomes, concluding that the most effective programs focused on engaging patients during inpatient services and connecting the patient to increased utilization of community-based services. The programs seem more effective for patients of medical disease versus mental health issues.

Care coordination models are also included as components of Medical Home models. Care coordination is described in that context as providing patient care oversight and support by aligning community agencies, hospitals/emergency facilities, and medical specialist through communication and information connectivity to ensure accountable patient care. Through the Medical Home model, care coordination can follow the patient through each care transition. This means that information must accompany the patient care event and precede and send information timely to record and transmit proper patient care information.

Antonelli et al. described how a busy pediatric practice used care coordination to serve children with special care needs within a practice setting.[27] These patients were complex and totaled 11% of the empanelled patients while consuming 25% of the total encounters during the measurement period. They required staff time four times longer than typical pediatric patients. Coordination of care included processing referrals, consulting with schools or educational programs, and oversight for psychosocial issues.(Antonelli, McAllister, Popp, & Fund, 2009)

A significant aspect of healthcare reform is transforming the delivery of care from a volume-based, per-visit (fee-for-service) model to a value-based model. In this new, value-based world, health care providers take a significant role to "manage" a population and all services rendered to their patients, regardless of multiple organizations participating in their care, with the goal of ensuring quality, cost-effective care is experienced by all their patients.

> *INSIGHT:* Value based care is blind to the number of patients requiring medical intervention. The expectation is that each patient receive quality cost-effective treatment plans. Successful treatment of patients is dependent upon providers managing populations respecting that the patient may receive out-of-network intervention. Managing the patient in all transitions is critical to evaluate and manage the total cost-of-care. Quality care must be measured in all transitions. As organizational networks solidify, providers must work together and minimize any negative effect of out-of-network visits.

As ACOs become effective, they oversee and are responsible for the total care of their population, and each individual member. The member may receive care from more than one healthcare organization, yet the ACO is charged to "coordinate" the care, reduce overall cost of care, and preserve the quality rendered. Because of the focus on value, resulting "challenges" of quality and assumption of the risk of the cost of care, an integrated network that decides to become a risk-bearing accountable care organization will logically strive to use medical professionals within its own organization to manage these challenges and overcome barriers to refer within the group.

Review of the Literature

Published studies show mixed impacts on health outcomes and costs from care coordination, and there is little agreement on the design of care coordination interventions. When managing patients and populations, interventions that studies have shown to be effective include: transitions of care (care when transferring between healthcare facilities/professionals), medication management, patient engagement and self-management, education (community based programs), patient direct outreach, intermediary between patient and provider, and social support. A common theme running through the studies is that careful attention to detail is required to cost-effectively manage each patient and the overall population.

The available literature on care coordination is characterized by an array of models, processes and activities focusing on differing populations with varying complexity, all being defined as care coordination. A common element of these models is the intent to arrange disparate aspects of the care of a patient or groups of patients in an organized fashion. The entire continuum of care is represented in the literature on care coordination including variations in age, condition, health concern, population, provider and setting. The unit of care may be static or spread out over time it may refer to the organizing of activities during a single episode of care and setting or between settings such as in transitional care, or it may refer to a set of activities over sequential and differing episodes of care. The coordination may be during acute care or it may refer to care of those with chronic disease in ambulatory, home, or other settings.

In an attempt to study whether care coordination improves the quality of care and how it affects cost, the Balanced Budget Act of 1997 mandated the Secretary of Health and Human Services conduct and evaluate care coordination programs and their effect on cost in the Medicare fee-for-service settings.(U.S. Congress, 1997) Eligible fee-for-service Medicare patients (primarily with congestive heart failure, coronary artery disease, and diabetes) who volunteered to participate between April 2002 and June 2005 in 15 care coordination programs were randomly assigned to treatment or control (usual care) groups. Hospitalizations, costs, and some quality-of-care outcomes were measured with claims data for 18,309 patients enrolled through June

2006. A patient survey 7 to 12 months after enrollment provided additional quality-of-care measures.

Peikes et al. summarized the outcomes of the Balanced Budget Act of 1997 study of care coordination.(Peikes, Chen, Schore, & Brown, 2009) Only two programs (Mercy Medical Center and Georgetown) had favorable statistically significant treatment-control differences in hospitalizations and sizable differences (−9.3% and −14.0%, respectively) in Medicare expenditures and one of those was not viable for the long term. Many of the other programs showed improvements in quality of care or cost containment but not both, or the improvements were either not statistically significant or applied only to a segment of the population and not the entire study group. The authors suggest that the most effective intervention for care coordination may be a combination of an ongoing model with five components they found to be most effective, combined with a proven transitional care model to prevent hospital readmissions.

Comparing the two programs with the most positive results, with the 10 unsuccessful programs, Piekes et al. note five differences worth noting. First, both of the successful programs averaged nearly one in-person contact per month per patient. Second, these two programs had favorable effects on populations with average monthly Medicare expenditures in a middle range of approximately $900 and $1,200 (most of the other programs had populations with much higher costs and terminal stages of illness, e.g., class 4 CHF), whereas only 1 of the 10 unsuccessful programs enrolled a mix of beneficiaries with average Medicare expenditures in this range. This finding suggests that programs may need to target patients who are neither at too low a risk of acute illness and hospitalizations for the program to have effects, nor so seriously ill that it is too late for interventions to have an effect. Third, In both programs, treatment group members were significantly more likely than control group members to report being taught how to take their medications. Fourth, care coordinators worked closely with local hospitals, and in fact the successful programs were hospital-based, which provided the programs with timely information on patient hospitalizations and enhanced their potential to manage transitions and reduce short-term readmissions. Finally, care coordinators in both programs had frequent opportunities to interact informally with physicians.

Volland et al. presents a detailed overview of the emerging research evidence on two approaches to primary care for the chronically ill, and the patient populations that benefit from their different perspectives and approaches to care: transitional care and comprehensive care coordination.(Volland et al., 2012) They concluded that both approaches have yet to demonstrate success in reducing total health care costs, although certain components of the models are potentially cost-effective when included in comprehensive efforts to manage the healthcare needs of adults with multiple chronic conditions. Targeting the appropriate level of interventions for individuals based on their health profile, educational background, and knowledge of the healthcare system and other resources are key in the effectiveness of these approaches when it comes to health outcomes and cost.

The two models of transitional care that Volland et al. review the Transitional Care Model developed by Mary Naylor and the Care Transitions Intervention developed by Eric Coleman, have shown reduced re-admissions and costs. Although the two models differ in approach, both engage patients with chronic illnesses while hospitalized; follow patients intensively post-discharge (for four to twelve weeks); engage in medication reconciliation; use a transitional coach or team to manage clinical, psychosocial, rehabilitative, nutritional, and pharmacy needs; teach or coach patients about medications, self-care, and symptom recognition and management; and, remind and encourage patients to keep follow up appointments.

An example of a comprehensive care coordination program is ValueOptions, a national company that provides employee assistance, health and life coaching, healthy connections engagement centers, reporting, Medicaid management programs, work/life solutions, and telepsychiatry.(Maryland Department of Health and Mental Hygiene, 2013) This comprehensive care coordination program utilizes a health information system to automate the reporting and tracking of patient care. They employ predictive modeling and risk stratification to "manage" high-risk comorbid populations and develop a locally-based, multi-disciplinary team to assist with transitions of care for the individual patient. The individual (along with person-specific barriers) is the focal point of their program. Their patient outreach is tailored to the individual. Additionally, they engage providers to meet the individual requirements of each patient. This model exemplifies a common strategy for managing healthcare at the patient level.

A growing evidence base suggests services that address social factors with an impact on health, such as transportation and caregiver support, can make these new models of care more effective. Examining early evidence from seven innovative care models, each with strong social support service components, Sheir et al. note that the evidence suggests coordinated efforts to identify and meet social needs of patients can lead to lower health care use and costs, and better outcomes for patients.(Shier, Ginsburg, Howell, Volland, & Golden, 2013)

Similarly, Claiborne defines three care coordination models that incorporate social services: centralized team model, regionalized, and provider-based.(Claiborne, 2006) The goal of these models is to integrate bio-psychosocial interventions for specific at-risk patients. The activity occurs primarily by phone and can offer enhanced services such as transportation, and housing assistance. Care coordinators screen and assess for quality of life and health status, educate patients, organize referrals, screen for psychosocial issues, assist and problem solve service need, advocate patient entitlements through public and private services, crisis intervene for mental health, coach self-care practices and adherence to treatment plans, and monitor patient progress and care.

Gittell et al. studied coordination within health systems using established scientific work around organization theory, especially as it relates to organizational social capital.(Gittell, Seidner, & Wimbush, 2010) Organizational social capital has been shown to improve performance by enabling employees to access resources that are embedded within a given network and by facilitating the transfer and sharing of knowledge. The related topic of relational coordination identifies dimensions of relationships integral to the coordination of work that is highly interdependent, uncertain and time-constrained – all characteristic of health care. Their study of nine hospitals revealed that relational coordination leads to high performance work practices and improved outcomes. There are seven dimensions validated in their fieldwork that have since been validated in subsequent studies, including: frequent, timely, accurate, problem-solving communication, and relationships of shared goals, shared knowledge and mutual respect.(Gittell, 2011)

Mapping the Challenges of Care Coordination

The pace of change caused by economic pressures and health reforms require the ability to move nimbly to incorporate best practices in care delivery. Yet information about rapidly evolving system threatens to overwhelm, and the availability of information through the Internet, social media, and other avenues challenges the capacity of organizations to consistently remain abreast of new findings, new models, and innovations in health care delivery, and maintain a robust vetting process to decide which changes to adopt.

In a rapidly changing healthcare environment, many organizations recognize the need for a disciplined, theoretical framework. Having the framework ensures maintaining perspective in the face of a growing breadth and depth of innovations, novel care models, and other care coordination challenges, without compromising the need to remain flexible, take risks, and learn through successes and failures. Regularly returning to evaluate care coordination work and its challenges against a framework permits rapid cycles of change without losing sight of known components. This is particularly true where there is no agreed upon set of competencies or measures for care coordination. It also maintains a process, independent of the changing whims or biases of individuals.

Therefore, we believe it is not only beneficial, but necessary to connect the process of mapping the challenges of care coordination to a framework that provides the theoretical foundation and logic to the mapping. To that end, the work of Houdt et al. is particularly pertinent. Houdt et al. provided an overview of the current theoretical frameworks for care coordination and performed an in-depth analysis of all identified theoretical frameworks to clarify key concepts related to care coordination.(Van Houdt, Heyrman, Vanhaecht, Sermeus, & De Lepeleire, 2013)

In that study, the 2007 Agency for Healthcare Research and Quality (AHRQ) review of five care coordination frameworks is used as the benchmark for the identification of theoretical frameworks around care coordination and to show how theoretical thinking can enrich the study of care coordination. Houdt et al. then searched through the PubMed/Cochrane database and found seven other frameworks that had emerged between 2007 and 2010. Together with the five frameworks in the AHRQ study, an in-depth analysis was performed of all of the frameworks (n=12).

Houdt et al. identified 14 care coordination concepts in the analysis of the frameworks: external factors, structure, tasks characteristics, cultural factors, knowledge and technology, need for coordination, administrative operational processes, exchange of information, goals and roles, quality of relationships, patient outcomes, team outcome, and organizational or inter-organizational outcome. These key concepts are put forward by the authors as a means to facilitate the selection of a useful theoretical framework for developing, studying and evaluating care coordination strategies. Two of the twelve frameworks emerged as being the most comprehensive because they incorporate more of the key concepts when compared with the other frameworks: the Relational Coordination Theory for exploring care coordination within an organization and the Multi-level Framework which can be used to study care coordination between organizations.

The Multi-level Framework is relevant to a CIN because it proposes that organizational design shapes networks. Gittell et al. argue effectively that the same formal practices that give rise to effective coordination at one level can also be used proactively to generate effective coordination at other levels. By using the same organizational mechanisms within and between organizations, clinically integrated networks are strengthened resulting in greater quality and efficiency.(Gittell & Weiss, 2004)

The organization design practices described in the Multi-Level Framework are: cross-functional routines or protocols, information systems, functional boundary spanners and cross-functional meetings. Integration is also achieved through the use of control mechanisms including shared incentives, shared performance measures and supervision. In examining the organization design literature, Gittell notes that traditional organization perspective underestimates the autonomy of departments within an organization, while overestimating the autonomy of organizations from each other. However, the problems of achieving effective coordination both within and across organizations are comparable in that both require deliberate design interventions to creative effective networks for coordination.

The 14 key concepts identified in the theoretical frameworks analysis are mapped to care coordination challenges in the fishbone diagram (see Figure 8-1). This type of diagram was chosen because of its ability to illustrate the complexity of the topic and give clarity to the major themes involved. The fishbone is a scientific tool used to identify and clarify causes of an effect of interest.(Nelson E.C., Batalden, & Godfrey, 2007) This mapping facilitates the systematic exploration of the key concepts to consider while retaining the confidence of the foundation of the research process from which they emerged, the goal of such an analysis is to improving work in the organization. As the experience of care coordination grows, modifications to this model may emerge.

Figure 8-1. Care Coordination Fishbone Diagram

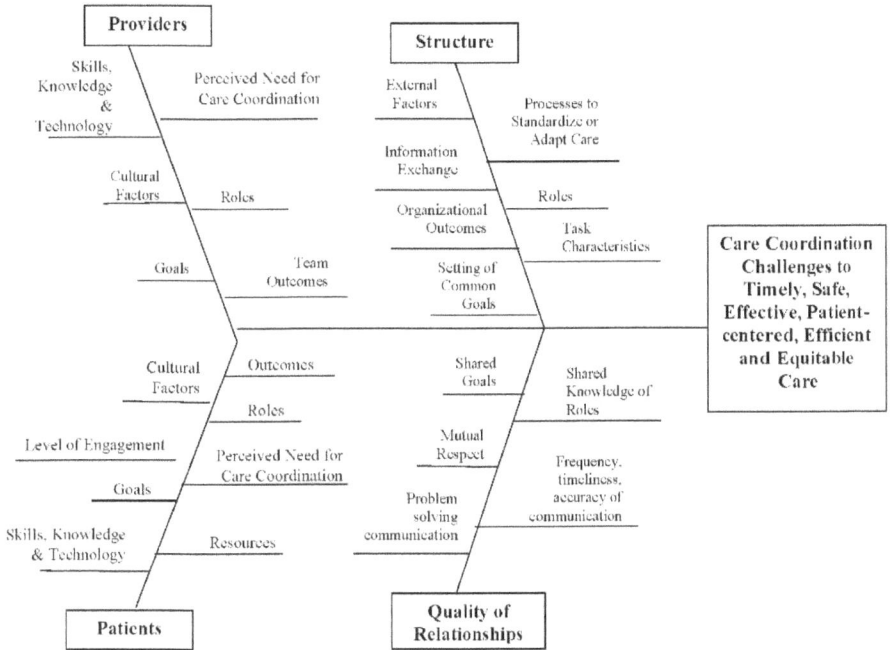

Care Coordination Challenges Fishbone Diagram

The fishbone diagram is comprised of the 14 key care coordination concepts grouped into four major categories (the big bones attaching to the spine), allowing them to be mapped to the care coordination challenges. Within each major category are multiple concepts which can be explored further for their contribution as specific causes of challenges to care coordination. In addition to serving as a mapping tool, the fish bone is an assessment tool and a model to launch improvement work. The exploration and potential improvement will depend on the characteristics and priorities of the organization interested in improving its care coordination. This mapping process is important as it provides a strategy with which to approach existing and future care coordination challenges.

As previously noted, the major care coordination concepts comprise the big bones and the various key concepts are listed on the smaller bones. Some of the key concepts recur in each of the major categories because the challenge is expressed differently within the category and merits a unique response. The major categories are: (1) structure, (2) patients, (3) providers, and (4) quality of relationships. Although the authors did not set out to do so, the categories resonate strongly with the four levels of the IOM redesign in the IOM Quality Chasm report described by Berwick: the organizations that house and support microsystems   and the environment of laws, rules, payment, accreditation, and professional training that shape organizational action (these two levels correspond to the 'structure' category); patients' experiences ('patients' category) and the "microsystems" that actually give care ('providers' category).

Structure

Under the concept of 'Structure' the following elements are clustered: external factors, processes to standardize or adapt care, information exchange, task characteristics, roles, goals, and outcomes. Aspects of structure considered when discussing care coordination challenges include the physical and organizational characteristics that support and direct care delivery. They also include the number of participating providers and provider organizations, their specializations and how they are grouped, the amount of information required to manage the care of the patient or patient group, and existing linkages between the entities. As noted previously, a major challenge that patients often unwittingly face in accessing health care is a formal system of care characterized by 'silos' because of poor linkages and accountability between and within entities. The Structure category is designed to address these challenges.

The 'External factors' linked with structure include national and state health policy, economic factors, dependency on regulations, and existing resources. Political leaders in health care must wisely steward revenue, develop appropriate policies and should remain connected to and learning from disciplines outside of healthcare. Historically, business acumen, policy and leadership theory, and organizational design have not been a part of medical, nursing or allied health curriculums. These cross-cutting dimensions should be infused through undergrad and graduate medical education to help address these challenges ingrained in healthcare. There should be recognition of the value of involving complementing expertise from outside healthcare, at both a macro and a micro level.

An example of an external factor is coding of patient care by physicians. How does a practitioner ensure that documentation and coding for reimbursement sufficiently and appropriately reflect the care being provided? An analysis of the fishbone for coding practices at the organization level may reveal a significant difference between national benchmarks and local utilization by providers. This may lead to creation of a 'cheat sheet' for major diagnoses coding, letting physicians understand the significance of diagnosis specificity, and appreciate the targeted and timely information at point of care. With the added reimbursement from proper coding of previously hidden procedures, it's possible that other activities physicians wish to do around patient care, but have been unable to afford, such as care coordination, may be within reach. Additionally, breaking the silos between hospital coders and provider is underappreciated, and ambulatory practices should consider embedding coders to improve diagnostic accuracy.

Evidence-based practice, another external factor, extends to the ability to monitor advances in other industries which may have relevance to healthcare. An example from the last decade in the published work of Provonost and Gawande is the recognition by open minded health care workers of safety principles which have been successfully developed and applied to improve processes in the aviation industry and can be applied in health care. The safety practices honed in aviation are now being modified, applied and scaled up in health care with compelling impact on patient outcomes.(Gawande, 2009; Provonost, September 3, 2013)

'Administrative operational processes' to standardize or adapt care are a part of the overall structure category. Impersonal methods involving standardized arrangements and minimal feedback, such as the rote application of guidelines, create an inflexible structure that may result in standardized care but not care that is adaptive or improving. Personal methods that communicate between individuals and teams with considerable feedback, and group methods with joint planning and decision making with maximum feedback, are methods which standardize or adapt care and improve processes.(Gittell & Weiss, 2004)

The 'Exchange of information' garners much attention in the literature. Different expectations about the information needed, lack of accountability, failure to provide timely and consistent information between providers and settings, lack of standardization based on best practice, and role clarification all are challenges involved in 'the exchange of information'. The relationship to outcomes is well documented, for example in the area of exchange of information about the patient's medication list between providers and settings, an area fraught with frustration and known lapses. Medication reconciliation is quickly becoming a standard best practice, shown to result in better quality care and reduced costs and errors.

The benefits of health information exchange and electronic record communication are assumed for the purposes of this chapter and can be read about in detail elsewhere. However, clinicians and administrative staff complain about the limitations and frustrations associated with electronic communication. Care coordination is affected by the capacity of practice staff to access and respond to information, and access should improve when it is sent electronically, but this is a capacity which varies considerably amongst practitioners. Different electronic record systems mean that 'work-a-rounds' have to be created for exchange of information, which is cumbersome and takes time. Maximizing existing EMR capabilities to overcome perceived difficulties requires more time and resources than many primary care practices can afford.(O'Malley, Grossman, Cohen, Kemper, & Pham, 2010) Overflow of information and "alert fatigue" has become common - just because a fax is sent or a record available does not necessarily help if there are multiple pages to read, or as one cardiac nurse said:

> 'We're glad to get the referral but to have to wade through all that paper when we are pressed for time – never mind find the medication list – is just too much.'

The concept 'Characteristic of the care coordination task' is placed within the structure of care coordination. Much could be written from an anecdotal perspective about the tasks associated with coordinating care at the point of service. As previously noted, a major challenge is the lack of standardization of the process of coordinating patient care, especially during transitions and across settings. The variability in skills needed and the lack of certainty in outcomes contributes to the lack of standardization.(Van Houdt et al., 2013)

Some tasks may seem simple but require maturity and/or knowledge on the part of the clinician for optimal results. For example, in the case of delegation of a follow up phone call to a patient following transition out of the hospital, if the information needed can be determined by a question as straightforward as: 'What transportation have you arranged for your appointment tomorrow?' one may have reasonable confidence in the information gleaned. Considerable experience is required, however, on the part of the clinician to gain rapport with the patient quickly through such a 'cold call', to know how to ask the question and be able to identify less obvious issues that may need to be addressed. The patient may have every intention of going to the appointment, but lacks the resources necessary to get there and feels ashamed to disclose the problem. A checklist of possible phrases to use may be helpful in bringing to light issues that may be more obvious in a face-to-face encounter.

Another task is the timely and pertinent documentation of care management and care coordination. Because it is a longitudinal activity, spanning multiple settings and involving multiple practitioners, the work and value of documentation is a challenge. How much detail is needed for providers? What level of information needs to pass from one entity to another? Does software incorporate 'tickler' systems or just-in-time workflow tasks?

Coordination of care activities take time. The time is difficult to quantify, the results difficult to connect to outcomes and therefore difficult to justify for reimbursement. Making phone calls to different agencies, closing loops between service providers such as referral sources or when making referrals, analyzing data to target interventions all take time, which is not embedded in a fee-for-service models of payment. With the advent of value-based purchasing and accountable care, the value of care coordination activities may increase as providers assume more risk for the outcomes.

Patients

The second care coordination concept category is 'patients.' Embedded in this category are the cultural factors pertaining to patients, the perceived need for care coordination, patient resources, level of engagement, patient knowledge of and use of technology, roles, goals, and outcomes.

To state the obvious: patients vary greatly in their health status, health literacy, available resources, engagement with the health care system and their (or their caregiver's) ability to manage care. With the degree of specialization in healthcare, clinical information about patients can be highly complex and involve multiple disease processes. Cultural factors that may be critical to patient choice and healing, such as attitudes, beliefs, preferences, family situation and values factor into their participation in the health care system. Gittell and Wiess note that clinical, social and administrative information is not easily codified for transmission amongst providers.(Gittell & Weiss, 2004) Care coordination as part of population management is challenged by the need to use limited resources wisely with as many patients as possible without losing the specificity that may be necessary to engage individual patients and build their capacity to self-manage health care.

The patient and family caregiver are typically the only common thread in all settings and by default have to coordinate their care.(E.A. Coleman, 2003 Apr; Eric A. Coleman & Berenson, 2004) A challenge is that they often lack the skills, knowledge, confidence or connection with the kind of health coaching that effectively does that coordination. As mentioned previously, many patients live with multiple chronic conditions, complex health care needs and functional limitations that require comprehensive care coordination. Challenges exist in effectively engaging them in their own care, leveraging resources, and incorporating best practices using technology. In care coordination, patient centeredness is a constant challenge and requires intentional, sustained patient feedback.

Patients may not even perceive the need for coordination. Even if they do understand the need for coordination and have the capacity to coordinate their own care, they may not be willing to take responsibility for coordination. As the administrator of one emergency department said,

> 'We the health workers have created this in the health care system: because we have done everything for them and kept them in a passive role we have fostered a generation of patients who do not expect to participate in their care; they expect to just be recipients of care.'

This speaks to the validity of role clarification and goal setting, not just among providers or healthcare organizations, but also between patients, their caregivers, and systems of care.

Providers

The key concepts clustered around the category of Providers overlap somewhat with the Patient category but are expressed differently: skills and knowledge, proficiency with technology, perceived need for care coordination, and roles, goals and outcomes. The coordination dimension to health care is sometimes recognized by providers as common sense, but may be perceived as near impossible to execute due to a system entrenched in episodic and setting-specific payment silos. The status quo and absence of precedence in doing anything different also contributes to a lack of expectation. A physician may express anger over a delayed hospital lab report while ignoring a lack of timely communication of results from other clinicians.

There is a lack of education and skill about the relevance of data, benchmarking and population management. Physicians also struggle with the challenges of running practices without formal business or leadership education. In one review of the literature, Stille et al. note that in order to effectively accomplish the tasks of coordination, physicians need training in building teams whose education and skills respond to the physicians' panel of patients and whose roles are clearly defined, especially for the sake of the patient's understanding.(Stille et al., 2005)

Providers have 'new initiative fatigue' and are rightly skeptical about the difference promised by the next change. On the other hand, there is a deep seated desire to be part of excellent work, and hope their efforts are not wasted in the pursuit of better health for patients.

Expectations or lack of expectations is an unfortunate phenomenon that erodes the edges of care coordination efforts. Providers do not expect to take responsibility for the patient in transition. Coordination mechanisms are well intentioned but generally are ad=hoc and seem to collapse when those involved in the process leave the system. Providers do not expect patients will be able to take responsibility for their personal health information or medication list nor do they expect communication from providers in other specialties and settings. Providers do not experience nor expect accurate and timely communication from others in the system, despite evidence related to improved outcomes with robust two-way communication. Clinicians work in parallel rather than collaboratively, which leaves patients at risk for disjointed, ineffective care.(Stille et al., 2005) Opportunities to standardize the referral process abound but without common goals and role clarification it is unlikely to happen.

One specialist noted,

'I have worked for 20 years in this system and what we are talking about is a culture change. Physicians have been historically very competitive and worked hard to hold on to their piece of the action and are very suspicious of each other. We have to change that culture so that we are on the same team for the sake of the patient. It will take a change in the culture.'[citation]

Clinicians in urgent care centers feel that community physicians do not respect them and feel they are treated disrespectfully, particularly by specialists. When ambulatory or ED settings reach out to primary care physicians they find it difficult to get past the gate keepers to speak with the physicians for effective hand offs and become discouraged in doing so. Clinicians in the community are ignored by the hospitalists who do not know them and are not incentivized to keep the loop closed.

It takes time, effort and persistence to disseminate evidence-based practice effectively. When clinicians have read the literature, return to school or participate in work groups, there is more awareness of best practices and of the need to work toward models that demonstrate better outcomes. The adage 'it takes seven times for an adult to hear something' was never truer than with the area of sustainable change in a health care system, working with providers. Providers are constantly pushed for time, balancing multiple agendas, and stressed about risk management. Consistent messaging over time as well as using principles of adult learning are just as important for the providers as it is for patients. Indeed, it is important to demonstrate with the providers what they are being challenged to do with patients.

Relationships

Quality of relationships is another major challenge for care coordination. Perceived status differences among caregivers, and between caregivers and patients, undermine and challenge effective communication needed in coordinating patient care. Status differences between organizations in the continuum of care, such as the traditionally higher status a hospital has over other providers in the community, has also posed an obstacle to care coordination across the continuum.(Gittell & Weiss, 2004)

Addressing high-performance work practices that foster relational coordination is an opportunity for improved organizational performance.(Gittell et al., 2010) This includes selection of employees that have not only the technical skills but also team building skills, mutual respect, cross functional conflict resolution abilities, participation in shared rewards, who can appreciate cross functional face-to-face meetings, and respect the role of boundary spanners.

Our experience has shown how fragmented the relationships may be, and includes limited collaboration that crosses organizational boundaries and was initiated because of specific shared goals, such as reduction of re-hospitalization rates. These experiences involved Medicare intermediaries or forward thinking hospital systems managing heart failure patients. A local collaborative between hospitals and nursing homes, for example, generated important work around the use of personal health records and patient responsibility for medication lists. However, it stalled at the execution phase because of lack of shared resources and the time and leadership required on the part of all the stakeholders to persist in development of a sustainable model.

Factors contributing to quality of relationships on the fishbone chart include roles and goals. The patient centered medical home, for example, focuses on roles and relationships between roles in primary care practice, leveraging relationships to improve outcomes. Improved organizational performance is influenced by shared goals, appreciation for the overall work process, understanding by network participants of their own tasks, the tasks of others, and how they relate to overall work processes. Having respect for the work of others encourages members to value those contributions and consider the impact of their actions, further reinforcing the inclination to act with regard for the overall work process. This web of relationships reinforces the frequency, timeliness, accuracy and problem-solving nature of communication, enabling participants to effectively coordinate the work processes in which they are engaged.(Gittell, 2011)

Disrespect is one of the potential sources of division among those who play different roles in a given work process. Occupational identity serves as a source of pride, as well as a source of invidious comparison. Gittell describes how members of distinct occupational communities often have different status and may bolster their own status by actively cultivating disrespect for the work performed by others. When members of these distinct occupational communities are engaged in a common work process, the potential for these divisive relationships to undermine coordination is apparent. By contrast, respect for the competence of others creates a powerful bond, and is integral to the effective coordination of highly interdependent work.

Sample questions in each of the key dimensions posed by Gittell contribute to the mapping of challenges in the area of quality of relationships and suggest directions for improvement. For example, if the work process being examined is the caliber of handoff communication that occurs as patients move between provider settings, the following questions can be posed to providers in the different settings:

- *Frequent Communication*: How frequently do people in each of the groups communicate with you about the patient population in transition between your facilities?

- *Timely Communication*: Do people in the groups communicate with you in a timely way about the patients in transition?

- *Accurate Communication*: Do people in the groups communicate with you accurately about the patients in transition?

- *Problem Solving Communication*: When a problem occurs with patients in transition, do the people in the groups blame others or work with you to solve the problem?

- *Shared Goals*: Do people in the groups share your goals regarding patients in transition?

- *Shared Knowledge*: Do people in each of the groups know about the work you do with patients in transition?

- *Mutual Respect*: Do people in the groups respect the work you do with patients in transition?(Gittell, 2011)

Making these questions open ended and the use of 'why?' may glean helpful information on which to base improvements.

The fishbone tool allows an organization to map the challenges facing successful operationalization of care coordination and explore their causes. The four major groupings: structure, patients, providers and quality of relationships reflect the major issues facing healthcare organizations in implementing care coordination.

The Recommended Care Coordination Model

Care coordination has a vital role within a clinically integrated healthcare organization. It is distinct from case management. Nevertheless, case management has a broad and varied role within an organization. The case manager in an inpatient department or ambulatory clinic works directly with the patient and physician (Primary Care Provider [PCP]) or specialist). The manager directly engages the patient with their care and services, educates the patient about disease management, facilitates solutions, and overcomes barriers that inhibit effective care. Many hospitals utilize case managers to assist with transfer to sub-acute facilities and follow-up after discharge. Larger organizations may use case managers to follow patient populations for specific disease prevention programs, to limit readmissions, etc. Many organizations incorporate case managers in their electronic home monitoring (telemedicine) to follow patients within a specific population to minimize disease complications and readmissions. For example, congestive heart failure patients can be transitioned home with scales and blood pressure monitors that are used to automatically send biometric values to case managers who monitor these patients' chronic disease and maximize ambulatory treatment efficacy. Case managers assist with discharge follow-up, and tailor medical service referrals to reflect the individual's needs. A common operational issue that distinguishes case management from care coordination is that once a patient is discharged the case manager no longer works with the individual, or continued contact is narrowly focused to the exclusion of other chronic diseases or healthcare issues.

Care coordinators, on the other hand, reinforce the culture of the integrated network and the inherent linkages they instill among physicians, hospitals, and skilled nursing facilities. Care coordinators, based at the corporate/enterprise level, do not necessarily have direct patient contact. Instead, they utilize patient-specific and population medical data to constantly oversee the attributed patients of the organization. Attribution is a function of a payer/employer identifying the PCP responsible for the patient. The PCP member of a clinically integrated network organization is interdependent with the other physicians, and therefore the collective patient population of all PCPs determines the population of the organization.

With the corporate/enterprise level care coordinator, information technology is utilized to effectively organize attributed patients based upon risk, care gap alerts, and transition status (for example between home, hospital, ED, urgent care), to focus resources of the enterprise, reduce barriers to care, and enable/encourage the local network provider to effectively manage the individual patient. When the local facility is unable to effectively assist an individual the care coordinator may assist directly. Care coordination facilitates enculturation of process standardization to more effectively serve patients within the population. Care coordinators reinforce, encourage, and monitor patient care using Information technology to monitor attributed patient care processes (standardized playbook adherence) through constant vigilance of reporting dashboards for patient care.

Care coordination has greater potential to be effective when clinical integration is fully implemented. Clinical integration uses evidence-based science to guide care of an individual patient and the greater population. Clinical integration allows all members of the healthcare team to utilize evidence-based guidelines, care transition requirements, healthcare metrics, and patient engagement requirements to effectively manage patients. Standardization throughout the organization allows for patient and population reporting to monitor and manage short and long-term medical issues/challenges facing patients.

The metrics used to follow quality, cost, and efficiency can be reported to organizational members with actionable data to guide patient level efforts. A "Playbook" that lists all payer required quality metrics, evidence-based preventative and chronic disease management, and minimal requirements for effective transition of patients between healthcare providers/facilities allows patients' data to be presented to care coordinators to guide institutional patient care with actionable communication with providers. The "Playbook" serves as the reference from which each practice can develop protocols and internal processes to allow all team members to function at their highest skill level, provide focused attention to high risk patients, and manage the population of patients with diverse care challenges. Effective local case management utilizing institutional evidence-based guidelines will allow increasingly more individuals to achieve improved health and system-wide care coordination monitoring processes and consequently will improve the health of the population.

Communication within the healthcare organization happens continuously to meet patient specific medical challenges. Population data is delivered monthly to allow the practice/facility level staff to focus local resources to make the most impact on patient health. For example, best practice dictates that if a patient is discharged from a hospital or emergency department, the patient needs follow-up by a physician within 7-14 days.

The following case study provides an example of how care coordination serves as an integral part of improving service delivery in the primary care setting.

Case Study: Primary Care Physician's Practice

This thriving independent primary care practice has multiple offices in a geographic span of 20 miles. This physician group leads the network's vision to transform healthcare to achieve the "Triple Aim". Recently as part of the CIN, this practice has been in the process of making an application to NCQA for Patient Centered Medical Home (PCMH) status. The Practice Manager has no prior experience in a PCMH model or precepts and was charged by the physician owner to lead the application process which she has done. Patient satisfaction surveys in the waiting rooms and the hiring of an APRN are two recent practice enhancements made to complete the application.

The PHO has monthly patient care meetings with each practice. The agenda includes: (1) response to previously identified issues, (2) identify new challenges, (3) review of the patient and practice population, (4) review of the active care plans of high risk patients, (5) review of the Playbook, and (6) evaluate the PCMH application progress. The meeting identified existing patients with high prospective risk, readmission risk, patients who had utilized the emergency department (ED) in the prior 12 months and the patients past due for prevention tests.

Two patients were brought to the attention of the practice physicians: one was a female patient who used the ED frequently (five times in the prior year due to ambulatory sensitive conditions). The Practice Manager made a note in the electronic medical record in anticipation of an already scheduled visit that month. At the next month's care coordination meeting she was able to report that the physician discussed the ED visits with the patient and developed a more appropriate emergency plan with her. Relevant to that plan, as part of its PCMH application, the practice had recently adjusted its after-hours telephone messaging system to encompass safe access options communicated for the patients. Care Coordination staff will continue to support the local practice's monitoring of this and other patient's appropriate utilization but the patient is now aware of her physician's recommendations for her evidenced based care which is an effective predictor of behavioral change.

The Care Coordinator also reviewed a 57 year old male listed on the inpatient report and identified to have a high prospective risk. He has a severe complex cardiac disease with significant loss of ejection fraction

(5% to 10%). During the past year, he had been an in-patient three times (total of 19 days), in observation twice, elective inpatient admission twice for procedures, and to the ED. In the month prior the PCP said that the patient had been non-compliant in the past with all aspects of care and recommendations related to medications, dietary restrictions and follow up and had not cooperated with the PCP. The PCP was extremely frustrated with the patient and considered that the patient might consider another physician.

The Care Coordinator had collaborated with the network's heart failure (HF) clinic to follow the patient after the current hospitalization as part of the care plan facilitating the patient to connect to the network. The care coordinator learned from the HF clinic that he had refused to use the facility in the past. During the hospitalization, the attending cardiologist requested that an HF clinic nurse see the patient and try to convince him to go to the clinic. One of the HF clinic nurses did go visit the patient making a personal connection and advised him of the benefits of the clinic and how it worked. The patient reluctantly agreed to go to the clinic and an appointment was set for five days after discharge. The Care Coordinator recommended specifying incremental goals with which the patient could be successful.

Despite skepticism of the staff and physicians, the patient kept his appointment. The HF clinic's goal was to prevent a 30 day readmission and successfully educate the patient about better dietary choices, medication compliance, and self-monitoring techniques to decrease his symptoms and improve the quality of his life while living with heart failure. He was also instructed about the importance of carrying a current medication list with him at all times and showing the list at each health care appointment. This was accomplished because the patient kept his follow-up visits to the heart failure clinic over a period of four months. His wife and physicians receive frequent updates allowing the family to participate and reinforce the patient to participate with the care plan. At times, he has been impatient and stated he wasn't coming back but he has returned for each visit so far, has successfully decreased weight and has not been readmitted in four months. For this patient, the appropriate setting for care was the HF clinic. The PCP and HF clinic are now working as a team leading to successful patient engagement.

Clinical integration improves the ability for the healthcare team to share data between members of the organization to effectively follow the patient. This case study illustrated how care mangers organize and arrange for the follow-up of each patient, while care coordinators validate organizational success to meet the follow-up requirements. When the system is challenged, care coordination quickly identifies the barriers and begins to effect organizational adaptation to assure patient and population care.

Care coordinators are presented population data detailing those who are at risk of disease complications. They communicate with PCPs and specialists to aggressively manage patients thereby reducing their overall risk. Additionally, care coordinators share with each practice location patients who have not met disease or preventative care measures and summarizes for the practice where their focus will be most successful. Ideally, communication with each practice location is continuous to manage individual patients and periodically to manage patient-centered groups. An example is the bundle of tests recommended at regular intervals for the organization's diabetic patients: LDL, urine, hemoglobin A1C, foot and eye exams. Using information systems and health data (e.g., electronic medical records, claims data, etc.) the practices can tailor their patient outreach to anticipate test needs and to close gaps.

When the patient requires medical service not offered within the network, or the patient utilizes non-network services, care coordination is vital to evaluate and monitor the quality and cost of that care to develop strategic organizational growth and manage the cost-of-care to affect organizational shared saving programs. Given the intra and inter-organizational healthcare opportunities described, one can begin to appreciate how complicated the Multi-Level Framework becomes.

Medical management is differentiated from services. Medical services are the face-to-face patient-directed healthcare events. These include the physician-patient visit/event, and other health care encounters such as radiologic study and counseling by a nutritionist. Medical services are rendered to each individual patient. Case management is a component of services offered directly to the patient. This is done locally as close to the patient as possible to insure that socioeconomic barriers are considered and factored into the individual care plan. The care plan may be developed by various numbers of healthcare professionals, but the plan respects the patient's desire for care. Case management coordinates resources and opportunities to uphold the care plan and assure the patient of its success. The plan updates with each healthcare contact and change in patient status.

Care of patients with chronic disease continues to demonstrate disparities with care provision. Less than 50% of diabetic patients have timely eye exams. Many diabetics fail to have an HgbA1c evaluated at least two times per year. Actual follow-up after hospitalization or emergency room evaluation within recommended time frames frequently are not completed and these realities continue to increase the cost-of-care. Using a "Playbook" construct reinforces expectation and allows for identification of care delivery concerns. Even though case management programs have been institutionalized for many years, readmission rates, patient-care follow-up, and disease management measures still remain national challenges.

Clinical integration can minimize failure to facilitate patient data portability, improves intra organizational communication, minimizes the cost-of-care by reducing redundant services, and facilitates the right care at the right time with the right resource. Table 8-2 is a sample from an organizational "Playbook" detailing the minimum recommendation for diabetic care. The sample illustrates the measured metrics to be reported, the evidence-based recommendations to care for a diabetic patient, and allows providers and their support staff to anticipate patient needs to demonstrate quality care.

Table 8-2. Playbook Recommendations for Diabetic Care

WHO?	WHAT?	WHEN?
Adults ages 18-	➤ Check at least once annually:	During

WHO?	WHAT?	WHEN?
75 years with diabetes mellitus	o LDL-C level (target measure is <100 mg/dL) o Urine micro albumin or macro albumin or treatment of nephropathy o Neuropathy screen or evidence of medical attention to existing neuropathy o Blood pressure (Target measure is <140/90) o Tobacco use status (Target measure is # non-users) o Comprehensive foot examination o Dilated eye exam by ophthalmologist/optometrist o Serum creatinine & calculated GFR o BMI ➤ Check HbA1c at least 2 times annually; target measure is <8% for most patients (2-4 times based on goal) ➤ Prescribe at least 2 generic diabetic medications with at least 80% days covered since first Rx ➤ Two or more face to face visits for diabetes ➤ CCD printed; includes action plan	measurement year During measurement year In previous 2 years In the previous 12 months Every visit
Adults ages 18-75 years with	Documented daily aspirin or	During the measurement

WHO?	WHAT?	WHEN?
diabetes mellitus and ischemic vascular disease	antiplatelet medication use (ACCEPTED CONTRAINDICATIONS: Anticoagulant use, Lovenox (enoxaparin) or Coumadin (warfarin) Any history of gastrointestinal (GI)* or intracranial bleed (ICB) Allergy to aspirin (ASA) *Gastroesophogeal reflux disease (GERD) is not automatically considered a contraindication but may be included if specifically documented as a contraindication by the physician. The following may be exclusions if specifically documented by the physician: Use of non-steroidal anti-inflammatory agents Documented risk for drug interaction Uncontrolled hypertension defined as 180 systolic, 110 diastolic Other provider documented reason for not being on ASA therapy)	year

Future

"Flooding the Triple Aim zone"

Healthcare organizations have institutionalized various models of care coordination and case management. Few detailed descriptions have appeared in medical literature. Clinical integration is more than a proposed vision or philosophy; it should be an organizational mission that adapts to the perturbations of healthcare reform. Growing evidence, Einthoven et al., suggests that greater organizational integration is associated with higher quality and efficiency (such as reduced mortality secondary to myocardial infarction).(Enthoven & Tollen, 2005)

The American Hospital Association defines clinical integration as needing to facilitate the coordination of patient care across conditions, providers, settings, and time in order to achieve care that is safe, timely, effective, efficient, equitable, and patient-focused.(American Hospital Association, February 2010) To achieve clinical integration we need to promote changes in provider culture, redesign payment methods and incentives, and modernize federal laws. Care Coordination is the adhesive within a healthcare network that promotes recognition for evidence-based medicine and utilization of standardized medical delivery accentuating patient/provider communication and compliance to individual care plans.

Larger organizations are more likely to use organized care management processes compared to smaller organizations. Additionally, independent physician associations (IPA) are twice as likely to use effective care management processes as small groups without IPA affiliation. Medical Services are the patient care events occurring in each member's facilities. The services are face-to-face and include office visits, consultations, inpatient admissions, emergency department visits, special nursing facility admission, etc. Medical management is a total approach to managing attributed population while facilitating and focusing efforts to achieve preventative health maintenance while addressing existing chronic disease issues of each patient. Several authors (Ahgren, Axelsson, and others) have described horizontal clinical integration as the services within a facility and vertical clinical integration as services provided at the organizational level to "manage" the population while empowering each patient care location to successfully manage their empaneled patients.(Ahgren & Axelsson, 2007)

The following case study illustrates how taking advantage of system-wide information systems, care coordinators monitor all patients attributed to the PHO and facilitate internal data analysis distribution to each practice and physician. The data specifically articulates the patients attributed, and provides actionable guidance for each practice to focus local efforts to manage those patients with high risk or significant risk change, over utilizers of emergent services, those recently admitted, and the list of patients needing preventative care. Additionally enterprise care coordinators assist the local case managers with direct patient outreach for highly complicated patients requiring additional personalization to achieve disease management.

Case Study: Primary Care Physician and Urgent Care

A 44 year old Type 2 Diabetic was identified in monthly data review of the PCPs attributed patients. The care coordinator flagged the patient as requiring closer attention because the Emergency Department (ED) was used six times within a year. The primary and secondary diagnoses for the ED visits were all ambulatory sensitive. The Care Coordinator contacted the PCP who was unaware of the patient's history of ED visits, having not been consulted or given feedback by the ED. The last scheduled appointment for this patient was three months prior and he had been a 'no show'. He had last come for an appointment eight months before and then had been a 'no show' a month later. The patient had not responded to phone call reminders from PCP's office.

After reviewing the risk data, system utilization data, and overdue care alerts, the care coordinator purposefully contacted the PCP to review the patient's medical challenges. The PCP verbalized frustration because the patient seemed unengaged. The PCP reviewed patient data (from various sources including insurance claims). After discussion with the PCP, a care plan was developed.

The care coordinator attempted to engage the patient telephonically (voicemail), and after several attempts, direct patient contact was made (Friday afternoon). The care coordinator briefly described the care coordination program, the medical neighborhood concept, the need to maintain a relationship with a PCP, timely prevention testing, medication management, glucose management, less copays, and limited ED visits. The Patient was initially suspicious of the intervention, but willing to talk.

The patient said he was unable to go to the PCP during day because of his current work jobsite restrictions. He stated 'It's funny that you should call me - I ran out of my Metformin a few days ago. Twice I called my CVS and they got refills, first 10 pills and then 6 but I ran out a few days ago.' When the CVS Care Coordinator asked him about checking his blood sugar he responded: 'Well I left my glucometer at the place that I moved from so no - I haven't been checking that for a while.' He stated that he has continued to take his insulin. He had never been to an Urgent Care and denied knowledge that it is an appropriate alternative to the ED.

Through discussions with the PCP, the Urgent Care manager and the patient, he was redirected to the Urgent Care within blocks of his home and instructed to follow up with an appointment at the PCP within a week. The Urgent Care manager prepared the staff to receive the patient, and he was able to be assessed after work, received a prescription for his diabetic medication which he obtained at the pharmacy that night.

To reinforce the best practice transition protocol (described in the Playbook), the Urgent Care staff was reminded to communicate to the PCP about the visit. The patient was asked to make a follow-up appointment with the PCP. Finally, after one unavoidable cancellation and 2 phone calls from the PCP's practice and the Care Coordinator, he was seen by the PCP. Because he needed a glucometer, one was provided (supplied by a local vendor) during his follow-up visit.

Subsequently, new patient care alerts Indicated additional testing was past due (past due 25 months: LDL-C, HbA1c). When the Care Coordinator requested to the HbA1c and LDL results, the PCP noted to his surprise that he did not have them and was going to have the patient come to get the script and go to the lab. The Care Coordinator recommended electronic orders to Quest and a call was made to the patient to get the lab tests done. The patient was happy to go directly to the lab and avoid an extra copay. The next day he did go to the lab. The labs, which were abnormal, were available during the next follow-up PCP appointment for review.

In summary care coordination will:

1. Utilize patient and population data analysis to effectively promote preventive care.

2. Utilize data to manage chronic disease.

3. Utilize data to achieve payer quality and utilization requirements.

    a. Readmission

    b. ED utilization

    c. Ambulatory sensitive conditions

4. Coordinate system-wide patient management with payers.

    a. Coordinate care coordination activities to maximize patient outreach

        i. Collaborate with disease management activities provided by insurers

5. Strategically communicate with members of the clinically integrated network to maximize location specific activities to achieve practice-level success.

Figure 8-2 illustrates how clinical integration focuses on clinical outcomes, patient experience and engagement, and utilization of services. In the proposed model, a clinically integrated network must consider each of these components as distinct entities that continuously interact and are not "managed" in silo. Current case management models focus on patient engagement with limited attention to outcome and cost. The reason that case management is well accepted is that healthcare organizations strengths predominate by provider directed care to a patient/customer. The case manager will filter outreach according to facility immediate disease/service strategies. In a functioning clinically integrated organization, the focus is not facility-based championed by local stakeholders, but population-based for the attributed patients to the whole organization. Care coordinators work with each member of the organization to enculturate standardized patient care initiatives with respect to preventative and disease management, transition of care observance, and agnostic payer quality initiatives.

Care coordination actions significantly contributes to a clinically integrated network's success to achieve the "Triple Aim". CMS and other leading organizations repeatedly report that five to seven percent of the population consumes a large proportion of healthcare resources. These actions allow the network to operationalize population management to reduce the risk of the most complicated patients while addressing the needs of each patient within the population.

Health information technology is a vital component to arm care coordinators with the data necessary to achieve the stated goals. Additionally, the health information technology pulls data from disparate systems into meaningful reports necessary to effectively manage a population served by a clinically integrated network. Clinical outcomes and transparency will determine which organizations successfully adapt to healthcare reform. Successful organizations are able to use technology to evaluate quality care, manage chronic disease, and anticipate care gaps. Healthcare organizations will increasingly need to meet patient expectation and provide professional quality care. Ultimately, public reporting of organizational success achieving competitive levels of quality will reinforce patient engagement and assure that organizational patient attribution is preserved.

When considering a multi-level framework, an organization must be continuously aware of challenges external to the organization (public policy, national and state legislation, local competition). Structure within the organization is vital to withstand uncontrollable external perturbations. Healthcare organizations that achieve national recognition for achieving clinical integration excellence have the structure to manage a network that meets the "Triple Aim" goals. A network of medical providers exists in various levels of accomplishment and care coordination engenders the organizational culture of transformation. Change is not dictatorial but developed through relationships. Care coordination becomes the organizational glue that binds each member of the network to reach patient care goals that encompass the patient but affects the population at-large.

Authors such as Hernandez and Burns have differentiated the delivery of integrated healthcare through horizontal and vertical integration.(Burns & Pauly, 2002; Hernandez, 1999) Horizontal integration occurs when healthcare organizations consolidate and utilize economies of scale to benefit from purchasing, shared physical plant, shared capital, and spreading fixed costs over a larger base of operation. Additionally, a large organization could benefit from a wider patient base to make multiple service lines profitable. These organizations typically utilized the size to steer patients to a central "hub" facility. Unfortunately, realization of scaled savings has not been well demonstrated. Vertical integration attempts to provide patient care using multiple organizations seamlessly. The goal is to utilize providers and facilities that demonstrate cost-effective high quality care. Case management typically reinforces the horizontal approach to healthcare delivery, while care coordination's strength is to provide vertical care to the patient and population.

Vertical integration focuses on the care of a patient population. Successful vertical integration requires collaboration between aligned organizations and providers. Historically, horizontal care of the patient has not met with reduced healthcare cost. Consequently, public policy is driving alternative models. Intuitively organizations such as ACOs and PHOs that are responsible for populations of patients should be able to contain costs between economically competing entities to provide overall comprehensive patient care. These models of care, focused on population health and care coordination, should result in reductions in healthcare costs. Vertical care tested in small projects have demonstrated success.

Comparisons of facility charges are abundant in the literature. The cost of a hospital charge per day versus special nursing facility is dramatic. Greater attention is focusing on how to utilize the right setting to effectively provide patient care services. Unfortunately, barriers to using cost-effective settings are challenged by healthcare policy, and unfamiliarity with individual setting capabilities. Additionally, strong leadership is necessary to develop a clinically integrated network that offers significant options of patient care settings to advantageously provide quality cost-effective patient directed care.

Figure 8-2. Clinical Integration: A Vertically Integrated System

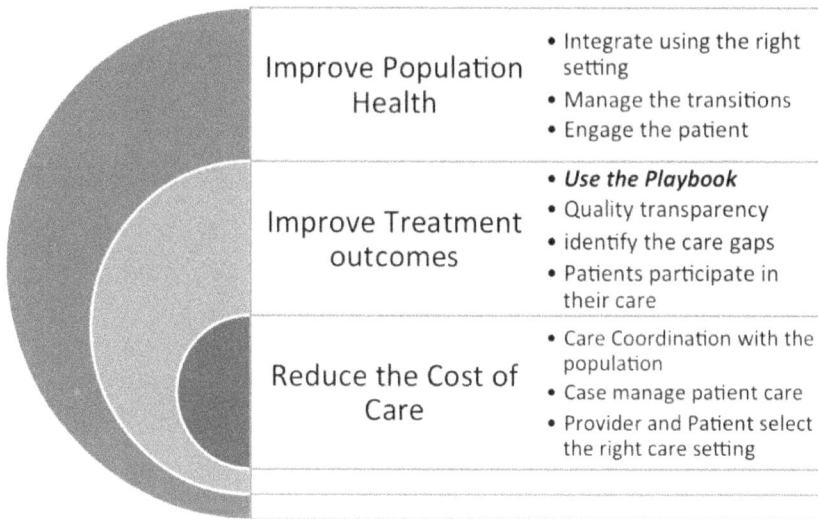

	Improve Population Health	• Integrate using the right setting • Manage the transitions • Engage the patient
	Improve Treatment outcomes	• *Use the Playbook* • Quality transparency • identify the care gaps • Patients participate in their care
	Reduce the Cost of Care	• Care Coordination with the population • Case manage patient care • Provider and Patient select the right care setting

Clinical integration in a mature healthcare system facilitates a patient to receive medical services in the right setting such as a patient's home, nursing facility, physician office, urgent care, or hospital. Clinical integration is the glue that combines medical services (direct patient care) and medical management (population health management) working in tandem to serve the individual without losing focus on the medical issues challenging the population. Clearly defining the roles of case management and care coordination as offered in the model provides a healthcare organization the vision to direct patient care to achieve the right care, at the right time, in the right setting, with the whole healthcare team participating in the care centered on the patient, respecting the patient, and affecting improved health of the population, one patient at a time and serving the whole population at large.

CHAPTER 8 DISCUSSION QUESTIONS

Study questions are provided for team building or class exercises. Answers for all questions are provided in Appendix C.

Question Number	Question
1	The fishbone diagram demonstrates the most common challenges facing an organization. How do you use the fishbone to meet the ever-changing organizational stressors that prevent high quality patient care?
2	What are the actionable features of the proposed care coordination model? How does it answer the Triple Aim?
3	Describe how the proposed care coordination model contributes to the goals of clinical integration.
4	Describe the difference between case management and care coordination.

ANSWERS TO CHAPTER 8 DISCUSSION QUESTIONS

1. *The fishbone diagram demonstrates the most common challenges facing an organization. How do you use the fishbone to meet the ever-changing organizational stressors that prevent high quality patient care?*

ANSWER:

The fishbone may be used to establish a baseline of the known contributing stressors to care coordination, unique to the organization. The fishbone has four major components: Provider, Structure, Patients, and Quality Relationships. Within each of those components or 'bones' are issues or processes that require organizational attention to achieve patient-centered, timely, safe, effective, efficient, and equitable care. Use the fishbone to clarify the cause and effect status of the challenges to care coordination unique to the organization. Opportunities for improvement can then be identified. Improvement work can proceed depending on decision making based on the organization's resources and priorities. This process provides a logical and sustainable strategy for continuous improvement.

2. *What are the actionable features of the proposed care coordination model? How does it answer the Triple Aim?*

ANSWER:

What are the actionable features of the proposed care coordination model? How does it answer the Triple Aim? The Triple Aim is high quality, cost effective care, centered on the patient. The model empowers every health care provider (irrespective of specialty) to provide coordinate case management directly with patient to take advantage of and enhance the provider-patient relationship. Care Coordination focuses on the population respecting evidence-based guidelines. Care coordination provides the provider with the homework to identify patients with risk, care gaps, and patients who are high resource utilizers. Care Coordination "empowers" case managers and provider staff to manage these individual patients. When quality is respected following national care guidelines and information is shared between providers then efficient use of medical resources occur. Quality care results in efficient use of medical resources that lowers current levels of cost. Patients are engaged in purposeful care coordination will have the opportunity to participate in the development of their care plans and consequently have personal stake in their care resulting in patient satisfaction.

3. *Describe how the proposed care coordination model contributes to the goals of clinical integration.*

ANSWER:

URAC's definition:

What is clinical integration?

Clinical integration is the coordination of patient care across conditions, providers, settings, and time to achieve care that is safe, effective, efficient, and patient focused. Smaller systems of care come together to form larger systems of care that broaden the purview of provider networks, ensuring dependable linkage between care settings and conforming enhanced coordination, and consistent use of evidence-based guidelines for managing patients.

Clinical integration requires providers to work together to share clinical data within a framework and network more expansive than a medical home, with the shared goal of rendering necessary care to patients in an efficient manner with the best possible outcomes. Successful clinical integration requires collaboration and coordination at all levels of the network, and URAC's Clinical Integration Accreditation sets the framework for the type of collaborative environment that controls costs, ensures quality, and improves health outcomes.

4. *Describe the difference between case management and care coordination.*

ANSWER:

Care coordination services are delivered primarily at the enterprise level while case management is delivered patient by patient at the local level. Case management directly engages the patient with their care and services, educates the patient about disease management, facilitates solutions, and overcomes barriers that inhibit effective care. Case managers assist with discharge follow-up, and tailor medical service referrals to reflect the individual's needs. Care coordination, on the other hand, reinforces the culture of the integrated network and the inherent linkages instilled amongst physicians, hospitals, skilled nursing facilities and ambulatory settings. Care coordinators, based at the corporate/enterprise level, do not necessarily have direct patient contact. Instead, they utilize patient-specific and population level medical data to constantly oversee the attributed patients of the organization and ensure gaps of care are closed. A common operational issue that distinguishes case management from care coordination is that once a patient is discharged the case manager no longer works with the individual, or continued contact is narrowly focused to the exclusion of other chronic diseases or healthcare issues, whereas with care coordiantion, the patient is always being evaluated for care gaps. See Table 8.1.

CHAPTER 8 HIGHLIGHTS

- The purpose of care coordination is to meet the Triple Aim.

- Care Coordination is a unique role and distinctly different than case management.

- Care Coordination is most effective within a clinically integrated network.

- The fishbone diagram mapping care coordination challenges facilitates analysis by organizations of the challenges and their causes for solution development.

CHAPTER 8 REFERENCES

Agency for Healthcare Research and Quality. (2011). Chapter 2. What is Care Coordination?: Care Coordination Measures Atlas. Retrieved November 23, 2013, from http://www.ahrq.gov/professionals/systems/long-term-care/resources/coordination/atlas/chapter2.html

Ahgren, B., & Axelsson, R. (2007). Determinants of integrated health care development: chains of care in Sweden. *The International Journal of Health Planning and Management, 22*(2), 145-157.

American Hospital Association. (2011). Hospitals and Care Systems of the Future. AHA Committee on Performance Improvement Report. Retrieved November 13, 2013, from http://www.aha.org/content/11/hospitals-care-systems-of-future.pptx

American Hospital Association. (February 2010). Clinical Integration – The Key to Real Reform. Retrieved December 3, 2013, from http://www.aha.org/research/reports/tw/10feb-clinicinteg.pdf

Antonelli, R. C., McAllister, J. W., Popp, J., & Fund, C. (2009). Making care coordination a critical component of the pediatric health system: a multidisciplinary framework.

Ball, T., Merry, M., & Verlaan-Cole L. (2013). Designing & Creating "Second Curve" Healthcare Systems. Retrieved November 13, 2013, from http://www.cicatelli.org/tpp/files/Designing%20%20Creating%20Second%20Curve%20Healthcare%20Systems1.pdf

Beasley, C. (2009). The triple aim: Optimizing health, care, and cost. *Healthcare executive, 24*, 64-66.

Berwick, D., M.,. (2002). A user's manual for the IOM's 'Quality Chasm'report. *Health Affairs, 21*(3), 80-90.

Burns, L. R., & Pauly, M., V.,. (2002). Integrated delivery networks: a detour on the road to integrated health care? *Health Affairs, 21*(4), 128-143.

Case Management Society of America. (2013). What is a Case Manager? Retrieved December 1, 2013, from http://www.cmsa.org/Home/CMSA/WhatisaCaseManager/tabid/224/Default.aspx

Chassin, M., R.,, & Galvin, R., W.,. (1998). The urgent need to improve health care quality: Institute of Medicine National Roundtable on Health Care Quality. *Jama, 280*(11), 1000-1005.

Claiborne, N. (2006). Effectiveness of a care coordination model for stroke survivors: a randomized study. *Health & Social Work, 31*(2), 87-96.

Coleman, E. A. (2003 Apr). Falling Through the Cracks: Challenges and Opportunities for Improving Transitional Care for Persons with Continuous Complex Care Needs. *American Geriatric Society, 51*(4), 549-555.

Coleman, E. A., & Berenson, R. A. (2004). Lost in transition: challenges and opportunities for improving the quality of transitional care. *Annals of internal medicine, 141*(7), 533-536.

Commission for Case Management Certification. (2013). FAQs about Case Management. Retrieved December 1, 2013, from http://ccmcertification.org/health-care-organizations/faqs-about-case-management

Committee on Quality of Healthcare in America, & Institute of Medicine. (2001) *Crossing the Quality Chasm. A New Health System for the 21st Century.* Washington, DC: National Academies Press.

Davis, K. (June 23, 2010). U.S. ranks last among seven countries on healthcare performance. Retrieved November 13, 2013, from http://www.healthcareitnews.com/news/us-ranks-last-among-seven-countries-healthcare-performance

Enthoven, A. C., & Tollen, L. A. (2005). Competition in health care: it takes systems to pursue quality and efficiency. *Health affairs-millwood va then bethesda ma-, 24*(5), 1383.

Gawande, A. (2009). *The Checklist Manifesto: How to get Things Right.* New York, New York: Metropolitan Books.

Gittell, J. H. (2011). Relational Coordination: Guidelines for Theory, Measurement and Analysis Retrieved November 17, 2013, from http://rcrc.brandeis.edu/downloads/Relational_Coordination_Guidelines_8-25-11.pdf

Gittell, J. H., Seidner, R., & Wimbush, J. (2010). A relational model of how high-performance work systems work. *Organization Science, 21*(2), 490-506.

Gittell, J. H., & Weiss, L. (2004). Coordination Networks Within and Across Organizations: A Multi-level Framework*. *Journal of Management Studies, 41*(1), 127-153.

Hernandez, S. R. (1999). Horizontal and vertical healthcare integration: lessons learned from the United States. *HealthcarePapers, 1*(?), 59-66; discussion 104-107.

Improving Chronic Care (ICC). (2013). Care Coordination. Retrieved November 23, 2013, from http://www.improvingchroniccare.org/index.php?p=Care_Coordination&s=326

Institute for Healthcare Improvement. (2011). Care Coordination Model: Better Care at Lower Cost for People with Multiple Health and Social Needs. Retrieved November 23, 2013, from http://www.ihi.org/knowledge/Pages/IHIWhitePapers/IHICareCoordinationModelWhitePaper.aspx

Keller, H. (2013). Helen Keller Quotes. Retrieved October 21, 2014, from http://www.successories.com/iquote/author/830/helen-keller-quotes/1

Macmillan Dictionary. (2013). Definition of Coordination. Retrieved November 13, 2013, from http://www.macmillandictionary.com/us/dictionary/american/coordination

Maryland Department of Health and Mental Hygiene. (2013). Comprehensive Care Management Program. Retrieved December 5, 2013, from http://dhmh.maryland.gov/bhd/Documents/ValueOptionsComprehensiveCare ManagementProgram.pdf

National Coalition on Care Coordination. (2013). What is Care Coordination? . Retrieved December 1, 2013, from http://www.nyam.org/social-work-leadership-institute-v2/care-coordination/

National Priorities Partnership. (2008). National Priorities and Goals: Aligning Our Efforts to Transform America's Healthcare. Washington, DC: National Quality Forum.

National Quality Forum. (2006). NQF-Endorsed® Definitions and Framework for Measuring Care

Coordination. from http://www.qualityforum.org/Home.aspx

National Quality Forum. (2010). Quality Connections: Care Coordination. Retrieved Novermber 17, 2013, from www.qualityforum.org

National Quality Forum. (2013). Effective Communication and Care Coordination. Retrieved Novermber 17, 2013, from http://www.qualityforum.org/Topics/Effective_Communication_and_Care_Coor dination.aspx

Nelson E.C., Batalden, P. B., & Godfrey, M. M. (2007). *Quality by Design.* San Francisco, CA: Jossey-Bass.

O'Malley, A., S.,, Grossman, J., M.,, Cohen, G., R.,, Kemper, N., M.,, & Pham, H., H.,. (2010). Are electronic medical records helpful for care coordination? Experiences of physician practices. *Journal of general internal medicine, 25*(3), 177-185.

Peikes, D., Chen, A., Schore, J., & Brown, R. (2009). Effects of care coordination on hospitalization, quality of care, and health care expenditures among Medicare beneficiaries: 15 randomized trials. *Jama, 301*(6), 603-618.

Provonost, P. (September 3, 2013). A Powerful Idea from the Nuclear Industry. Retrieved from http://thehealthcareblog.com/blog/tag/peter-pronovost/

Reuben, D., B.,. (2007). Better care for older people with chronic diseases: an emerging vision. *Jama, 298*(22), 2673-2674.

Robinson, K., M.,. (2010). Care coordination: A priority for health reform. *Policy, Politics, & Nursing Practice, 11*(4), 266-274.

Shier, G., Ginsburg, M., Howell, J., Volland, P., & Golden, R. (2013). Strong social support services, such as transportation and help for caregivers, can lead to lower health care use and costs. *Health Affairs, 32*(3), 544-551.

Slee, D. A., Slee, V. N., & Schmidt, H. J. (2008). *Slee's Health Care Terms* (Fifth ed.). Sudbury, MA: Jones and Bartlett's Publishers.

Stille, C. J., Jerant, A., Bell, D., Meltzer, D., & Elmore, J. G. (2005). Coordinating care across diseases, settings, and clinicians: a key role for the generalist in practice. *Annals of internal medicine, 142*(8), 700-708.

Balanced Budget Act of 1997 (1997).

Van Houdt, S., Heyrman, J., Vanhaecht, K., Sermeus, W., & De Lepeleire, J. (2013). An in-depth analysis of theoretical frameworks for the study of care coordination. *International journal of integrated care, 13*.

Volland, P. J., Schraeder, C., Shelton, P., & Hess, I. (2012). The Transitional Care and Comprehensive Care Coordination Debate. *Generations, 36*(4), 13-19.